Social Skill Scenes For Very Young Children With Autism

Maureen Mihailescu, MS

Copyright© 2011 Maureen Mihailescu
ISBN: 978-1-936509-07-2

No part of this publication may be reproduced, stored in a retrieval system, or transmitted in any form by any means, electronic, mechanical, photocopying, recording, or otherwise, without the written permission of the publisher.

Published by Windsurf Publishing LLC
        Greenwich, CT, USA

Library of Congress Control Number: 2011920606

Photography credits to Thinkstock

About This Book

    This book was created to help very young children on the autism spectrum gain better social awareness, confidence, and competency. Children with autism don't always recognize social opportunities around them while being in the presence of other children. They often need to be taught how to act and how to communicate appropriately with other children. Some children with autism might have severe language deficits while others talk well but the content of their language may not be appropriate for certain social situations or in need of improvement. This book was created for children who have these difficulties while approaching other children and communicating with them on a basic introductory level. Social scenes target behaviors that elicit asking other children their names, introducing yourself, making comments about what is happening at the moment, asking to play with someone, making additional comments, asking additional questions, and saying goodbye. These social scenes and question prompts are to be used with a therapist, parent, or teacher to practice these skills prior to generalizing in real and similar situations. It is important to know what the child is capable of doing now, called a baseline, and what we want the child to be able to do from the social scene practice. For example, can the child ask the first question, introduce himself or herself, make additional comments, ask additional questions without being prompted, and say goodbye appropriately? How much a child can do and where you wish the child to progress to is the goal of the intervention.

    In the back of this book there is data information and suggestions to record progress. I am also a believer that one should audio record, and at times video tape, children with these social communication needs to have an even more accurate idea of how their social language and behaviors improve. The number of appropriate responses, the spontaneity of responses, whether or not responses are prompted by someone or the child is able to respond by themselves, and how much effort is needed are important results to measure and observe.

    The goals here are not only better social communication skills but increased awareness of the different activities which children of these ages usually are active in. In addition to using the prompts in this book, one can talk about what the child or children in the pictures are doing, what is their body language, what might they be feeling, and so on. One can get as creative as one would like and expand upon conversation topics about interacting with other children and understanding them better.

    On the following page, I put a list of four words and definitions intended for the context of these exercises. These words should be discussed and examples should be acted out prior to beginning the social scene practice and role-play. They are introduce, comment, question, and goodbye. You might role-play with some of the child's toys, such as dolls or puppets, prior to beginning the exercises in this book. I also recommend using different scenes at the same time so as not to tire a child of a particular scene. It is best to use different scenes and go back to scenes rather than remain at the same scene over and over.

    If a child has extreme difficulty, continue to provide examples of appropriate social responses and keep trying to have the child at least repeat from examples until they respond on their own and begin to generalize with their own language skills. This expectation is very important. Also, when a child is producing, for example, two responses independently, keep requesting for more so as to continuously increase their communication competency abilities.

Maureen Mihailescu
M.S. in Psychology

Important Words To Know

Introduce - to say hello and tell someone your name

Comment - to say something about someone or something you see

Question? - to ask about someone or something you see

Goodbye - saying bye to someone when you are finished talking or being with them

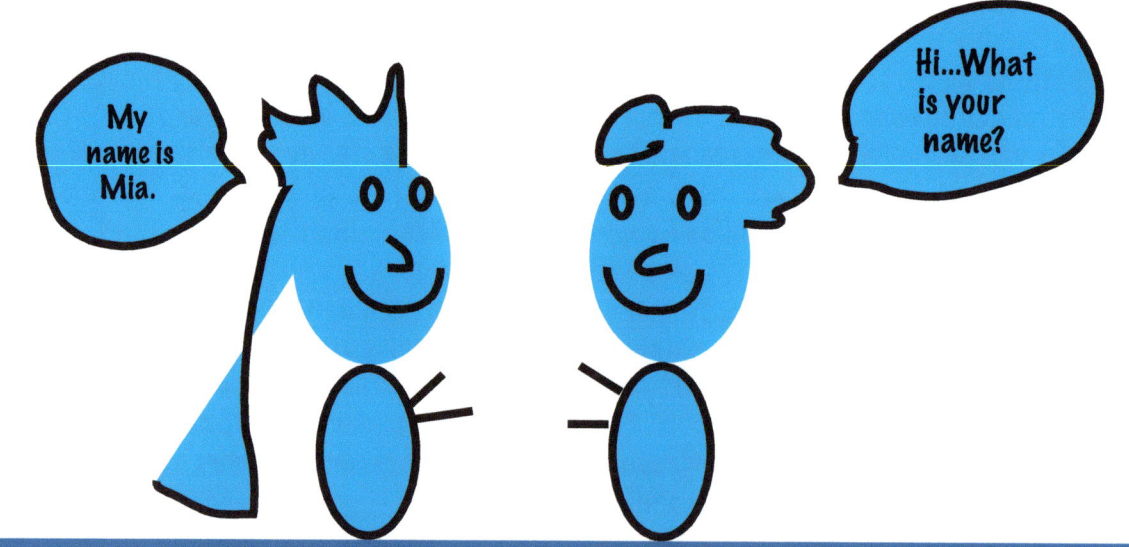

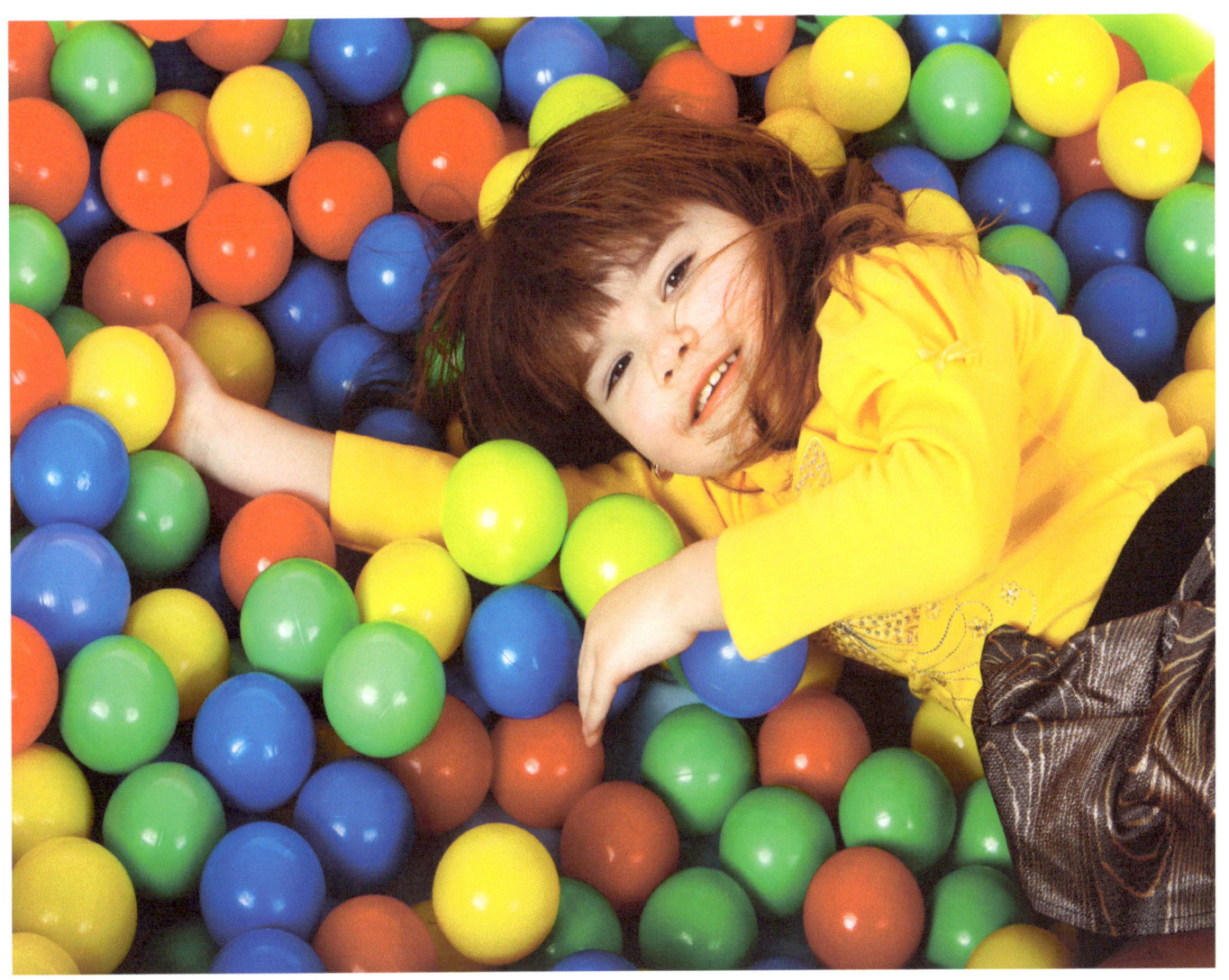

Social Scene 1: This girl is playing inside the kids ball bounce area. Let's pretend to...

Ask her what her name is...
Tell her your name...
Make a comment or ask a question about the ball bounce area...
Ask the girl to play with you...
Make more comments...
Ask more questions...
Say goodbye politely when your finished...

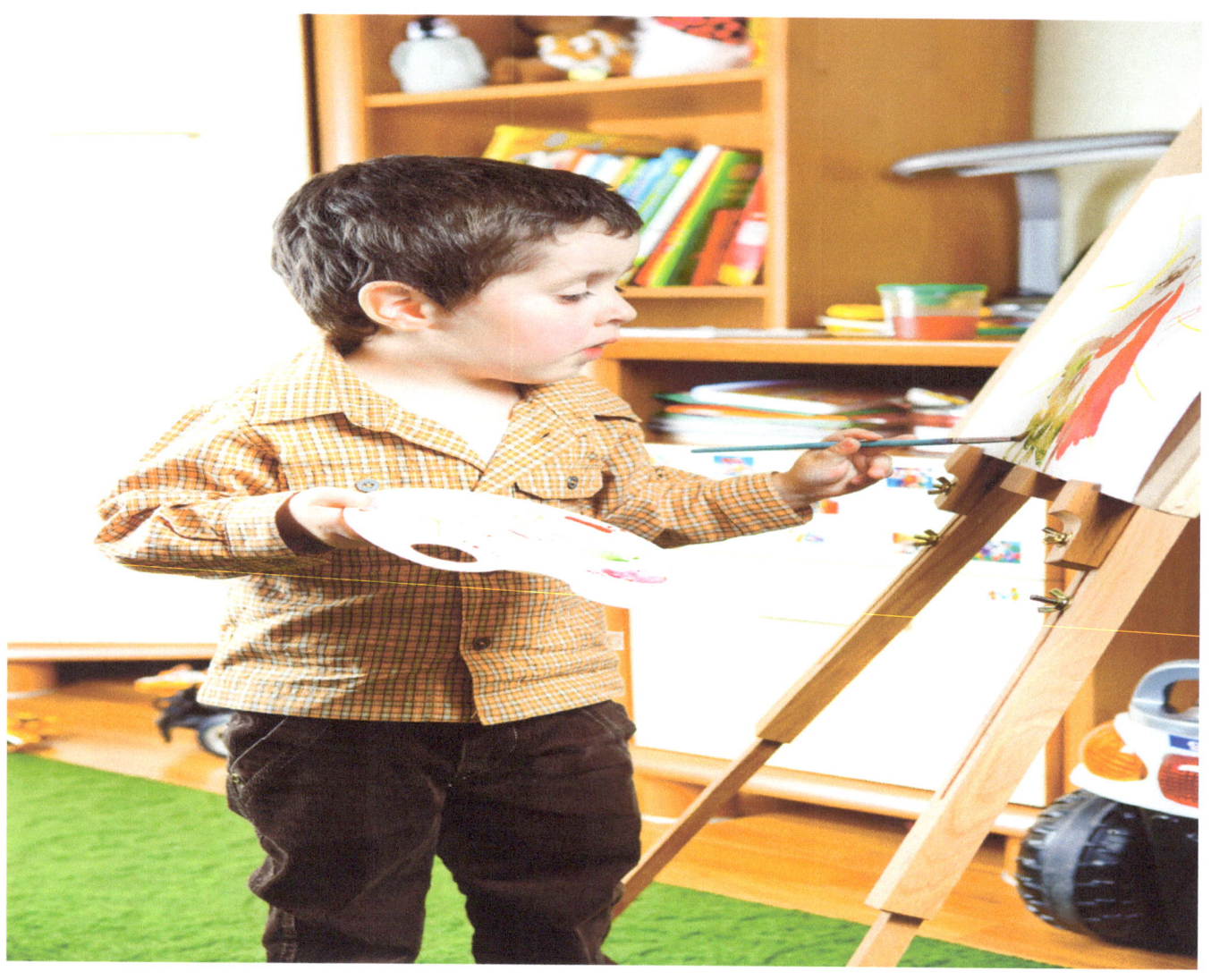

Social Scene 2: This boy is painting a picture with a paintbrush and paper at school. Let's pretend to...

Ask him what his name is...
Tell him your name...
Make a comment or ask a question about his painting...
Ask him if you could paint with him...
Make more comments...
Ask more questions...
Say goodbye politely when finished...

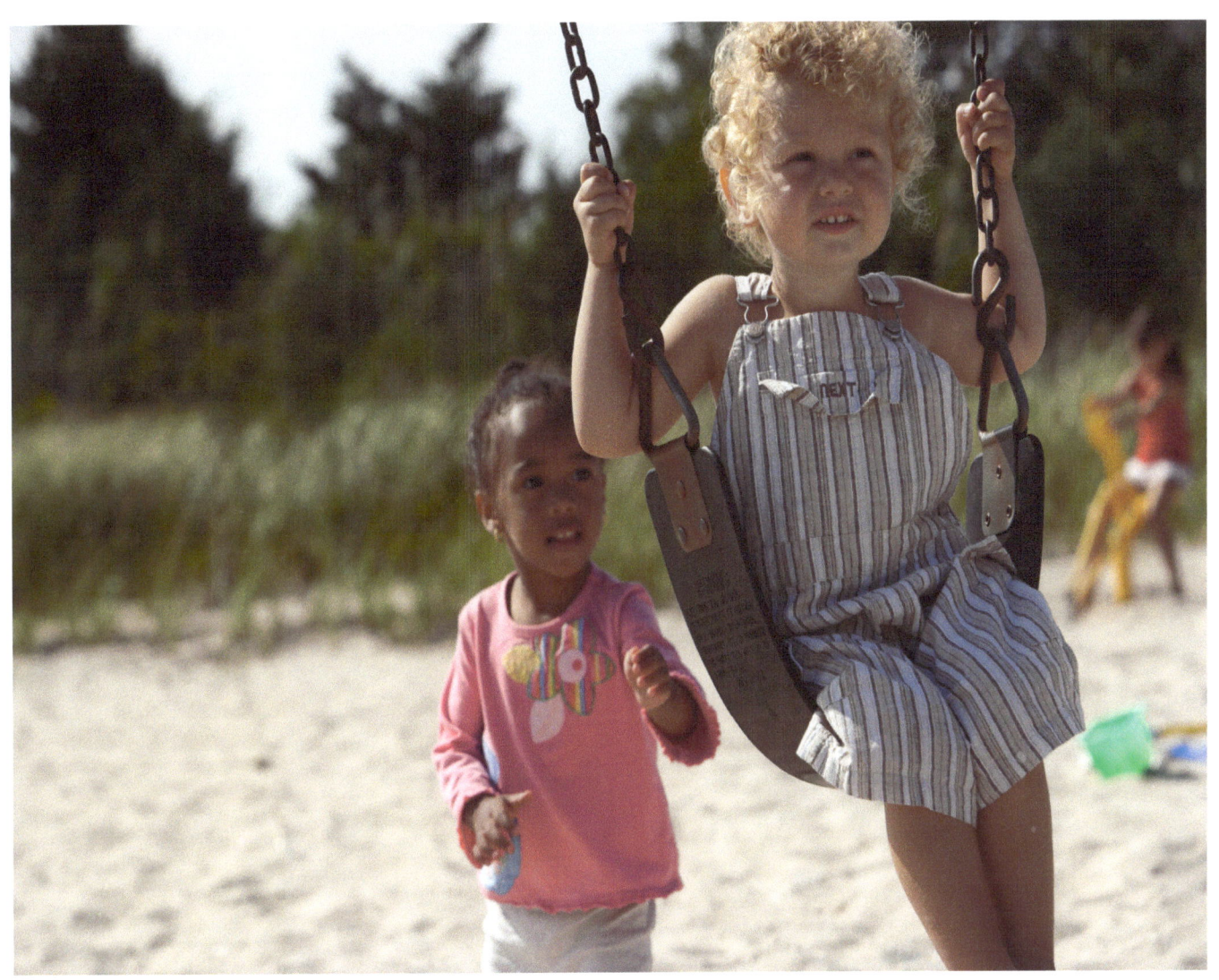

Social Scene 3: These two kids are playing with swings together at the park. Let's pretend to...

Ask them what their names are...
Tell them your name...
Make a comment or ask a question about the swings...
Ask them to play with you...
Make more comments...
Ask more questions...
Say goodbye politely when finished...

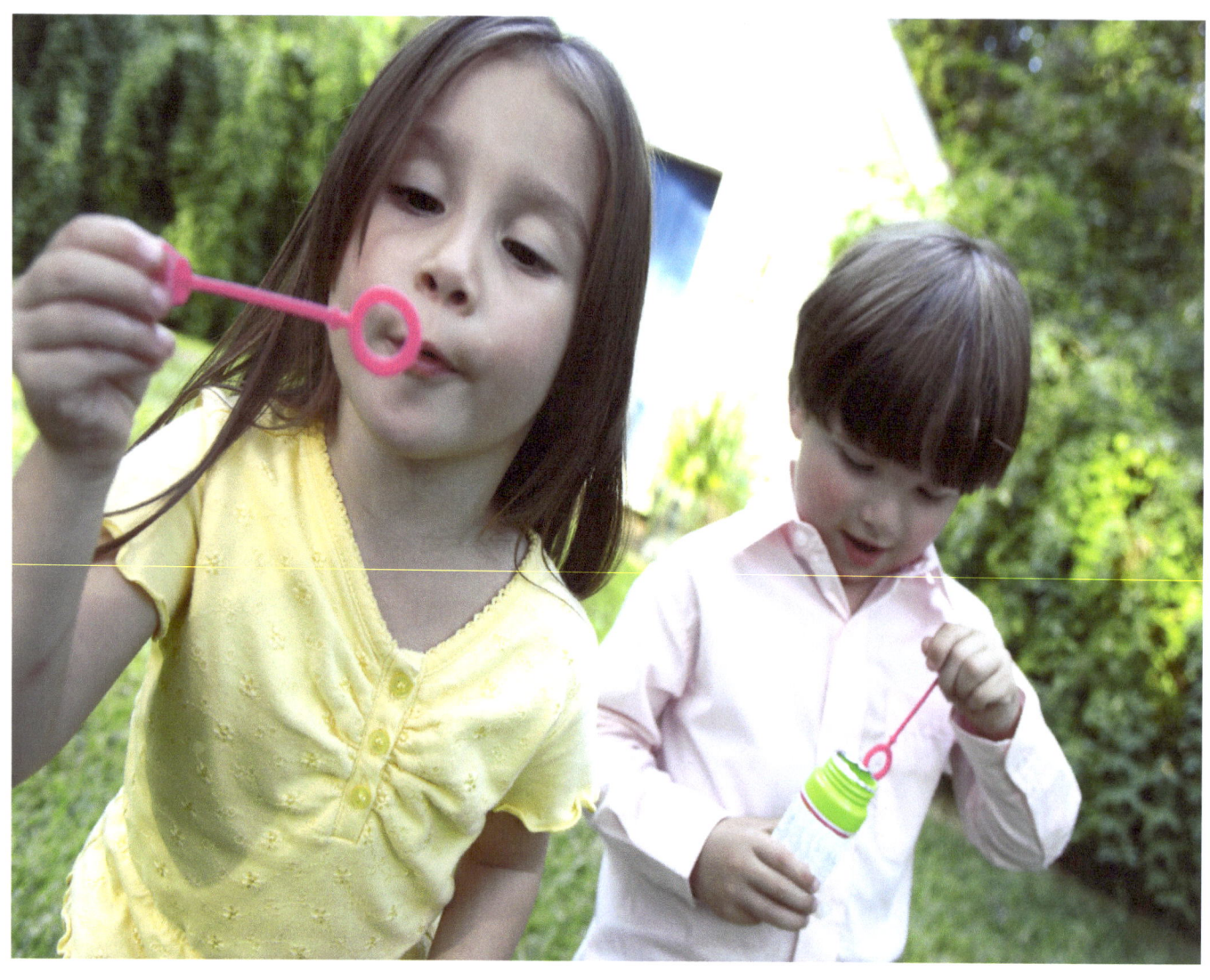

Social Scene 4: This boy and girl are blowing bubbles together at the park. Let's pretend to...

Ask them what their names are...
Tell them your name...
Make a comment or ask a question about bubbles...
Ask them if you could play with them...
Make more comments...
Ask more questions...
Say goodbye politely when finished...

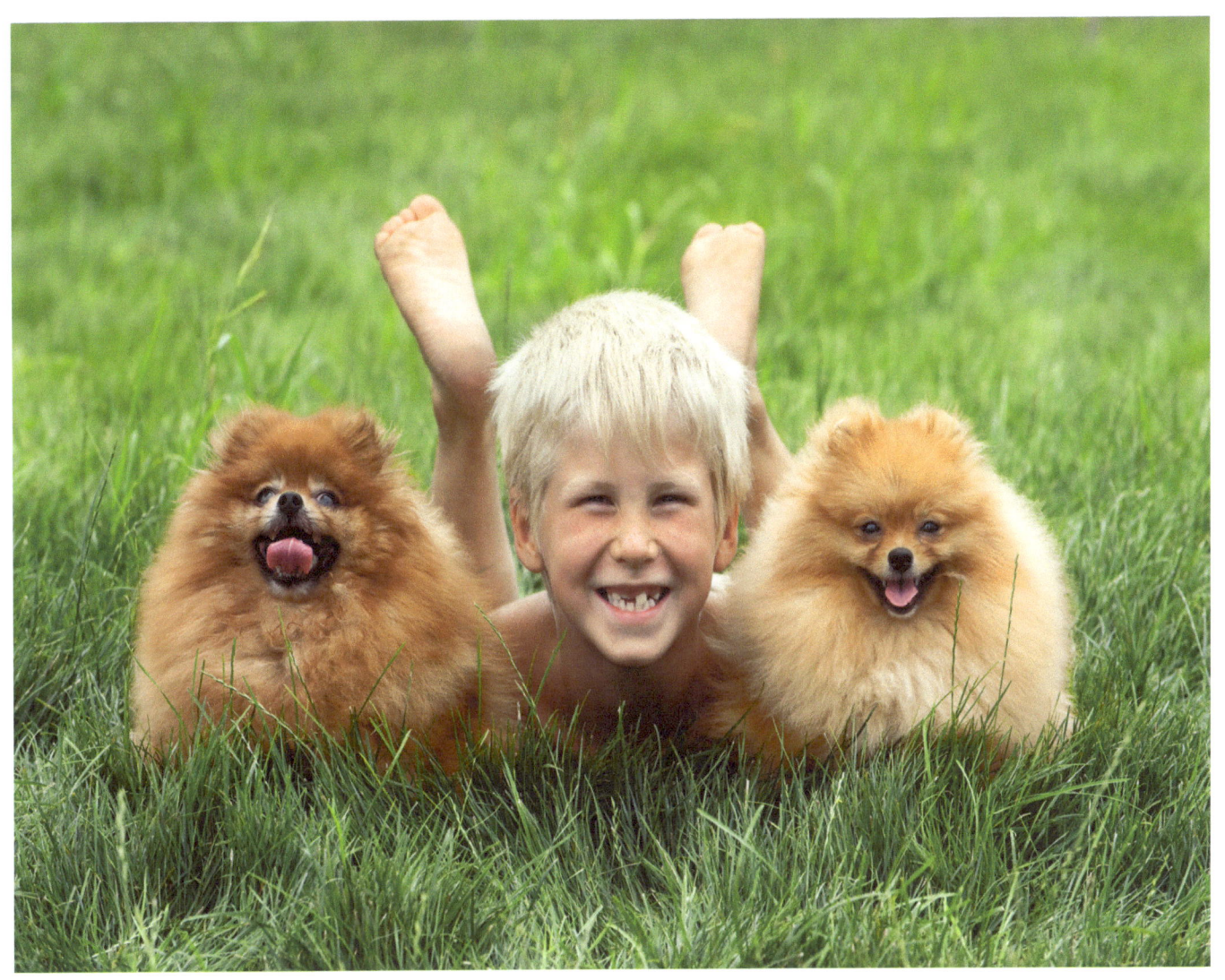

Social Scene 5: This boy is in the park with his two furry pet dogs. Let's pretend to...

Ask him what his name is...
Tell him your name...
Make a comment or ask a question about his pet dogs...
Ask him if you can pet or play with the dogs...
Make more comments...
Ask more questions...
Say goodbye politely when finished...

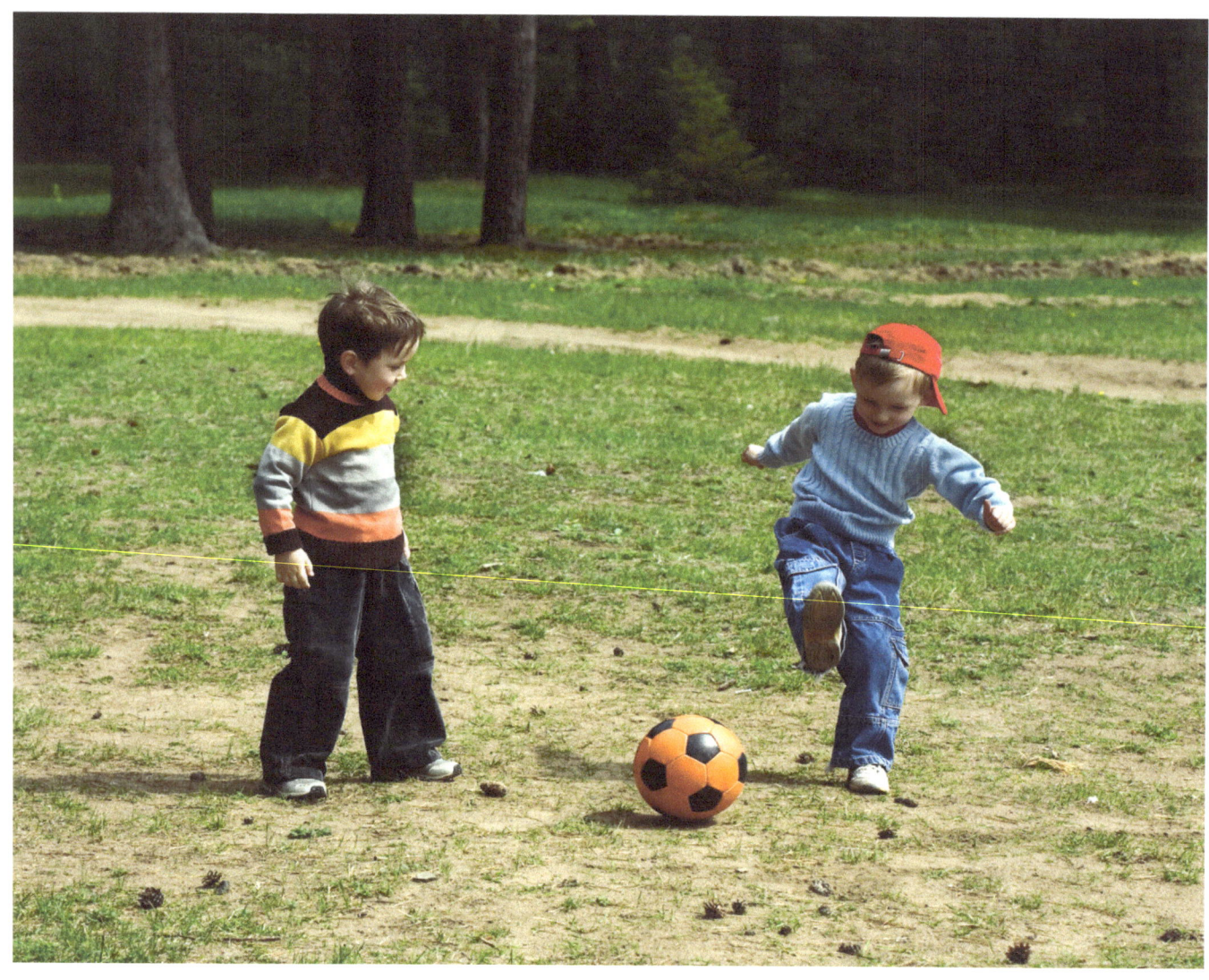

Social Scene 6: These two boys are playing with a soccer ball at the park together. Let's pretend to...

Ask them what their names are...
Tell them your name...
Make a comment or ask a question about the ball or playing...
Ask them if you could play with them...
Make more comments...
Ask more questions...
Say goodbye politely when you are finished...

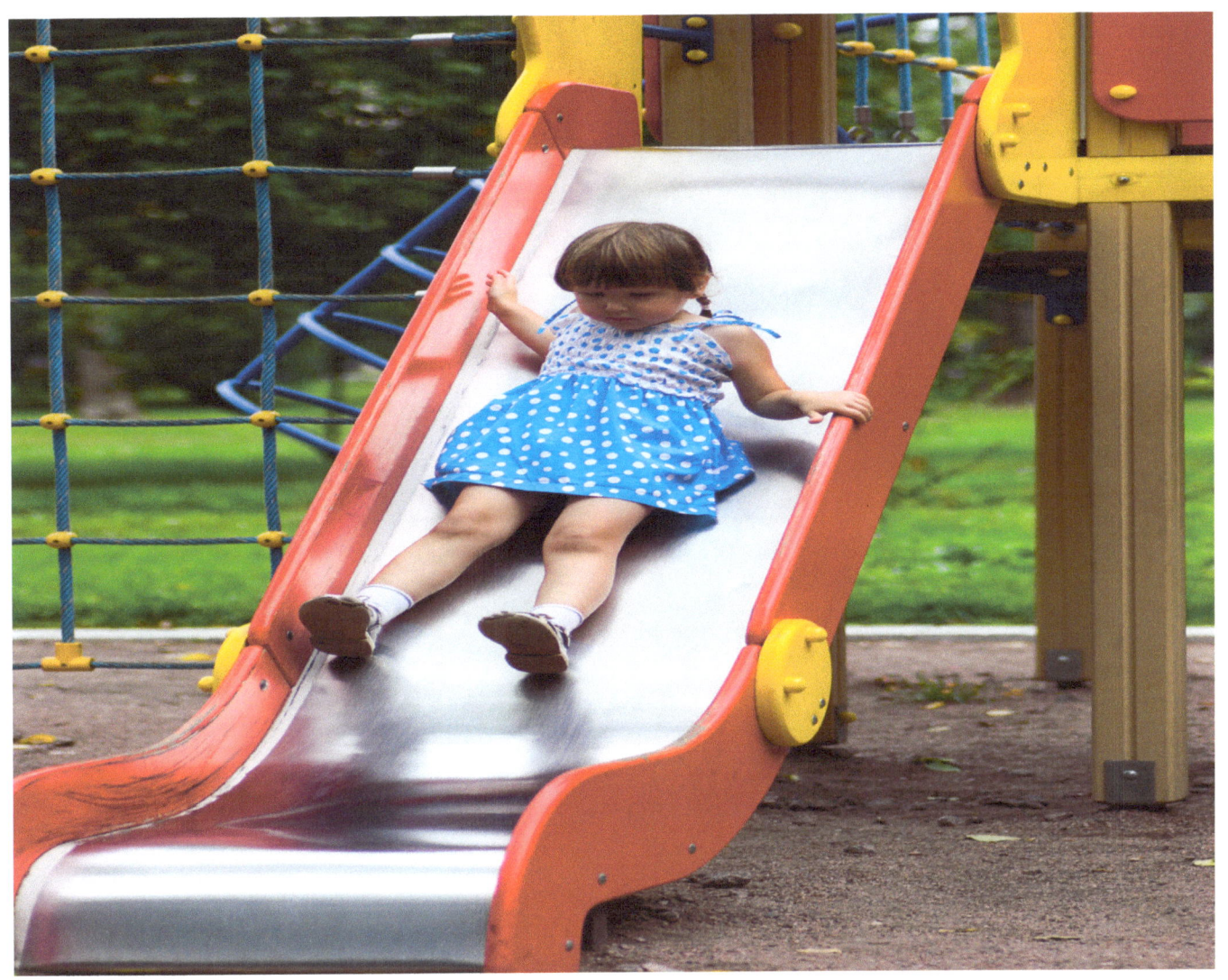

Social Scene 7: This girl is playing by herself on the slide at the playground. Let's pretend to...

Ask her what her name is...
Tell her your name...
Make a comment or ask a question about the slide...
Ask her if she wants to play with you...
Make more comments...
Ask more questions...
Say goodbye politely when you are finished...

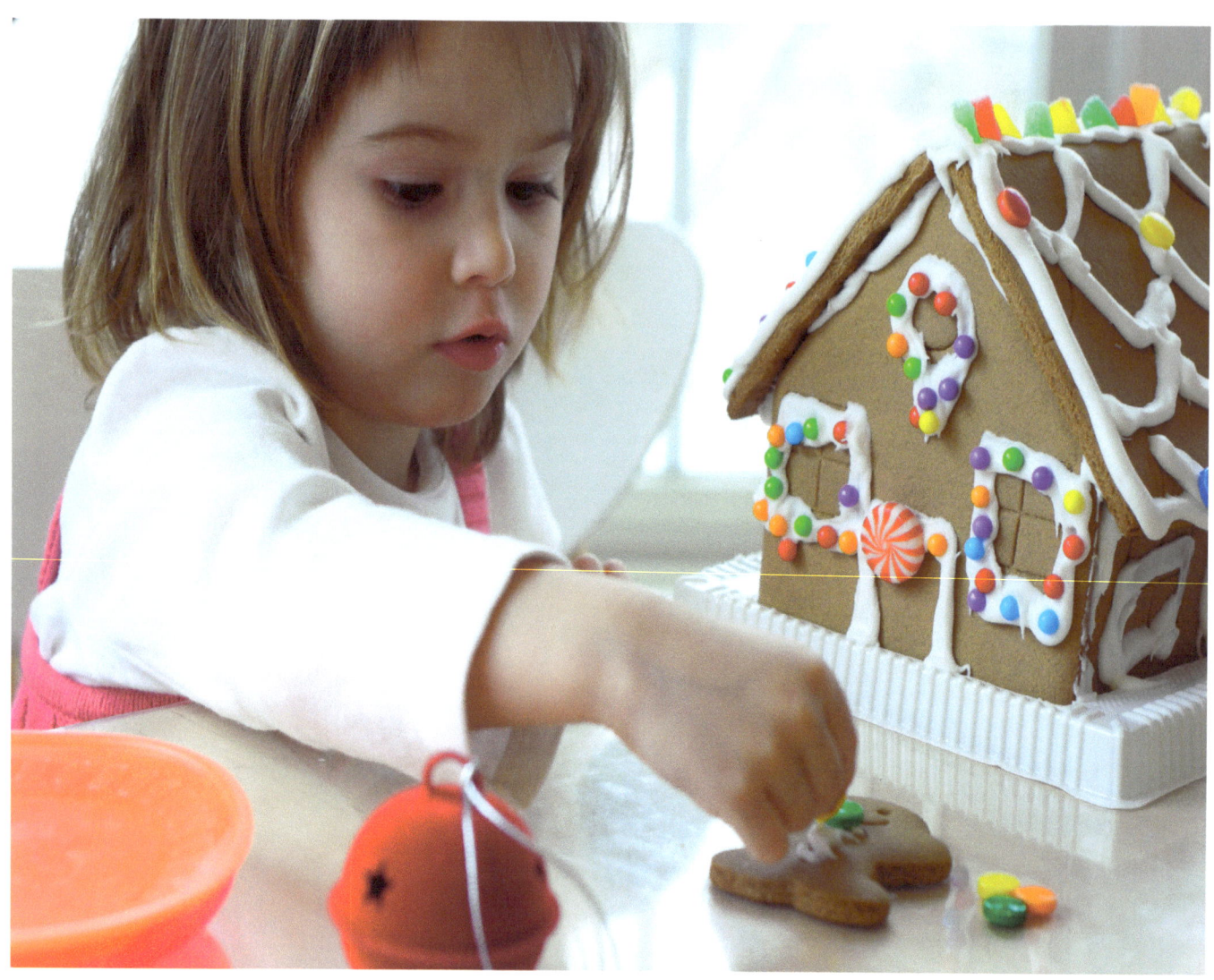

Social Scene 8: This girl made a gingerbread house and is now decorating cookies. Let's pretend to...

Ask her what her name is...
Tell her your name...
Make a comment or ask a question about her house or cookie...
Ask her if you could decorate some cookies too...
Make more comments...
Ask more questions...
Say goodbye politely when you are finished...

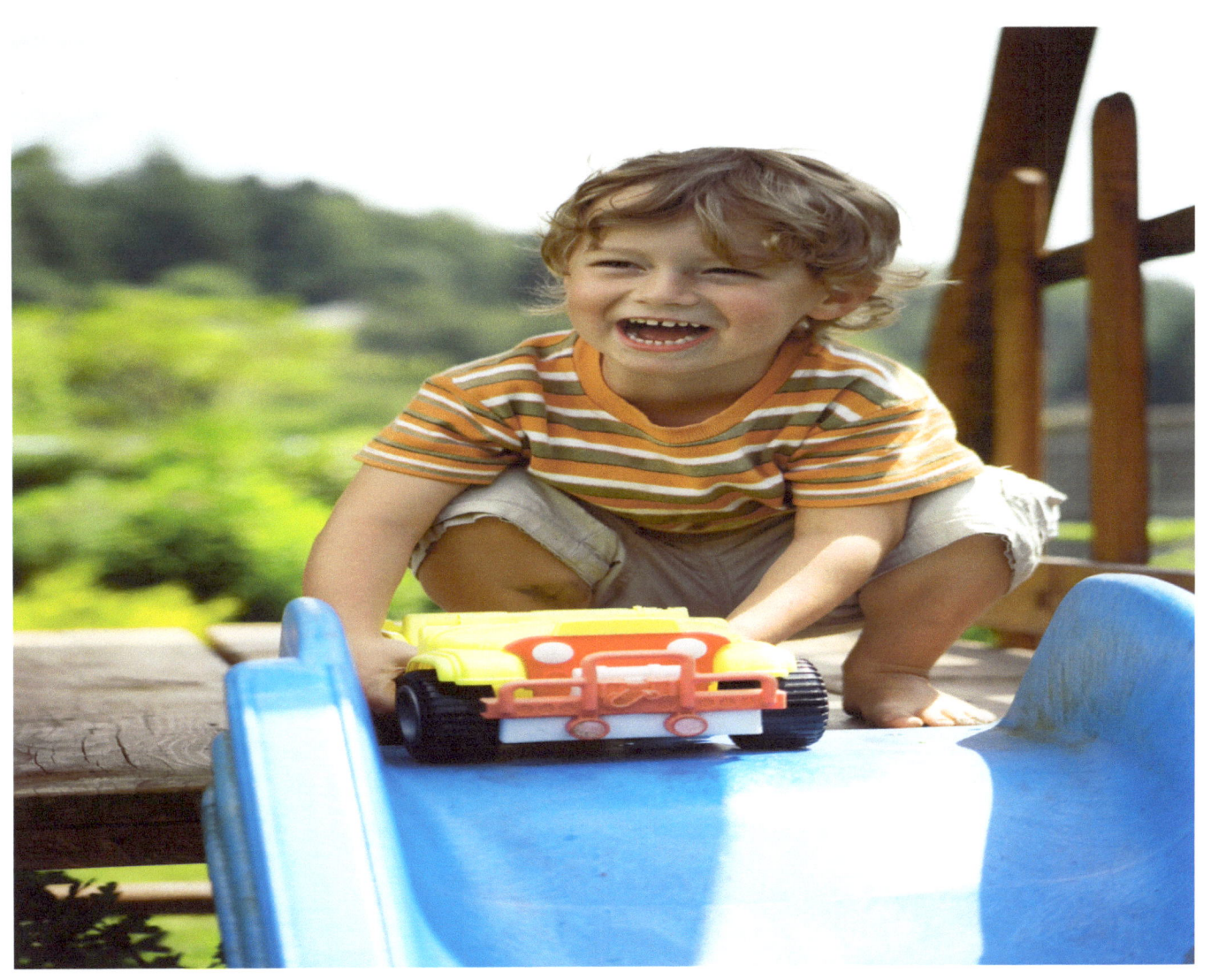

Social Scene 9: This boy is playing with a jeep at the playground. Let's pretend to...

Ask him what his name is...
Tell him your name...
Make a comment or ask him a question about his jeep...
Ask him if you could play together...
Make more comments...
Ask more questions...
Say goodbye politely when you are finished...

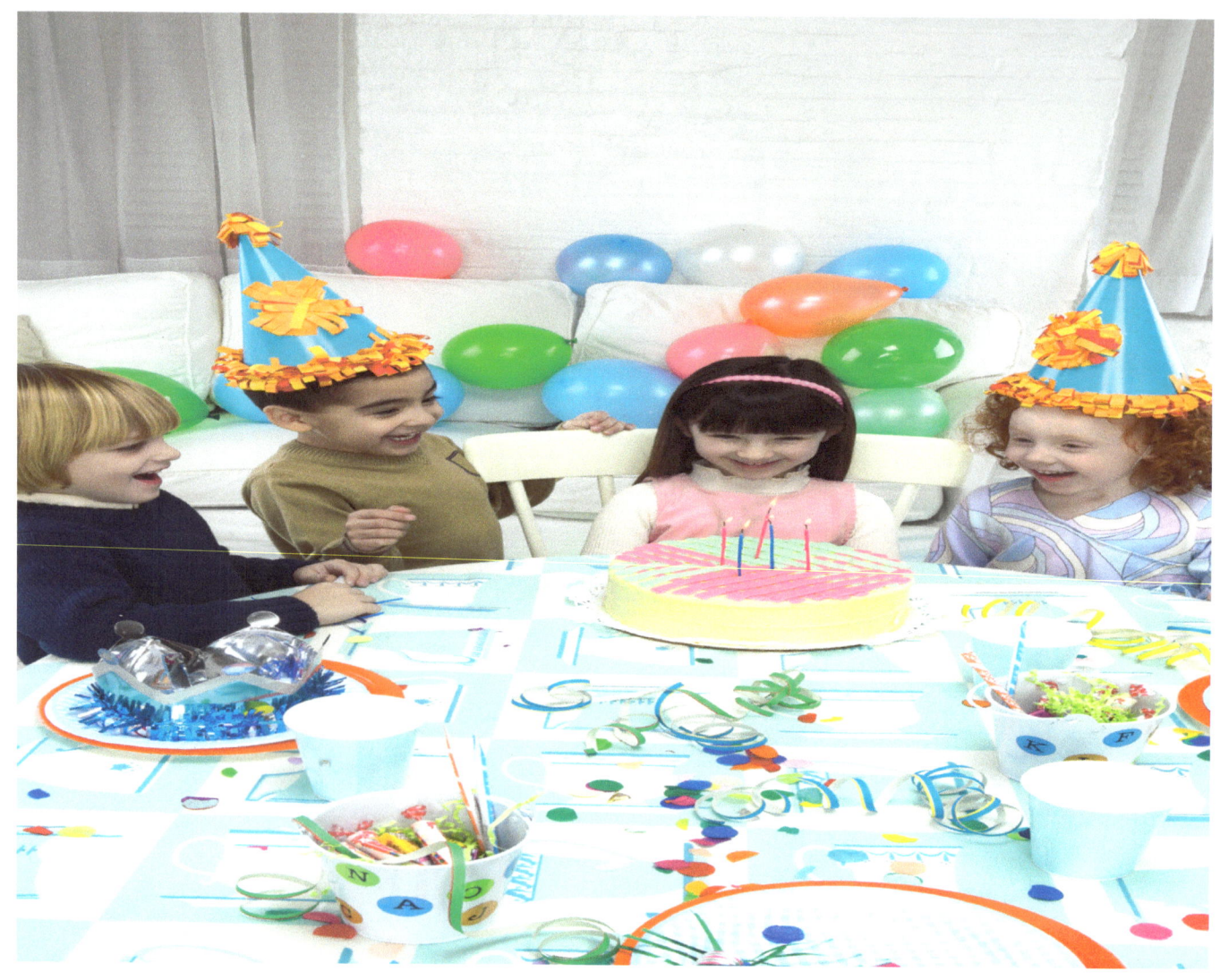

Social Scene 10: This group of children are enjoying a birthday party. You only know the birthday girl behind the cake. Let's pretend to...

Ask the other children what their names are...
Tell them your name...
Make a comment or ask a question about the party...
Ask if they will play a favorite game of yours...
Make more comments...
Ask more questions...
Say goodbye when you are finished...

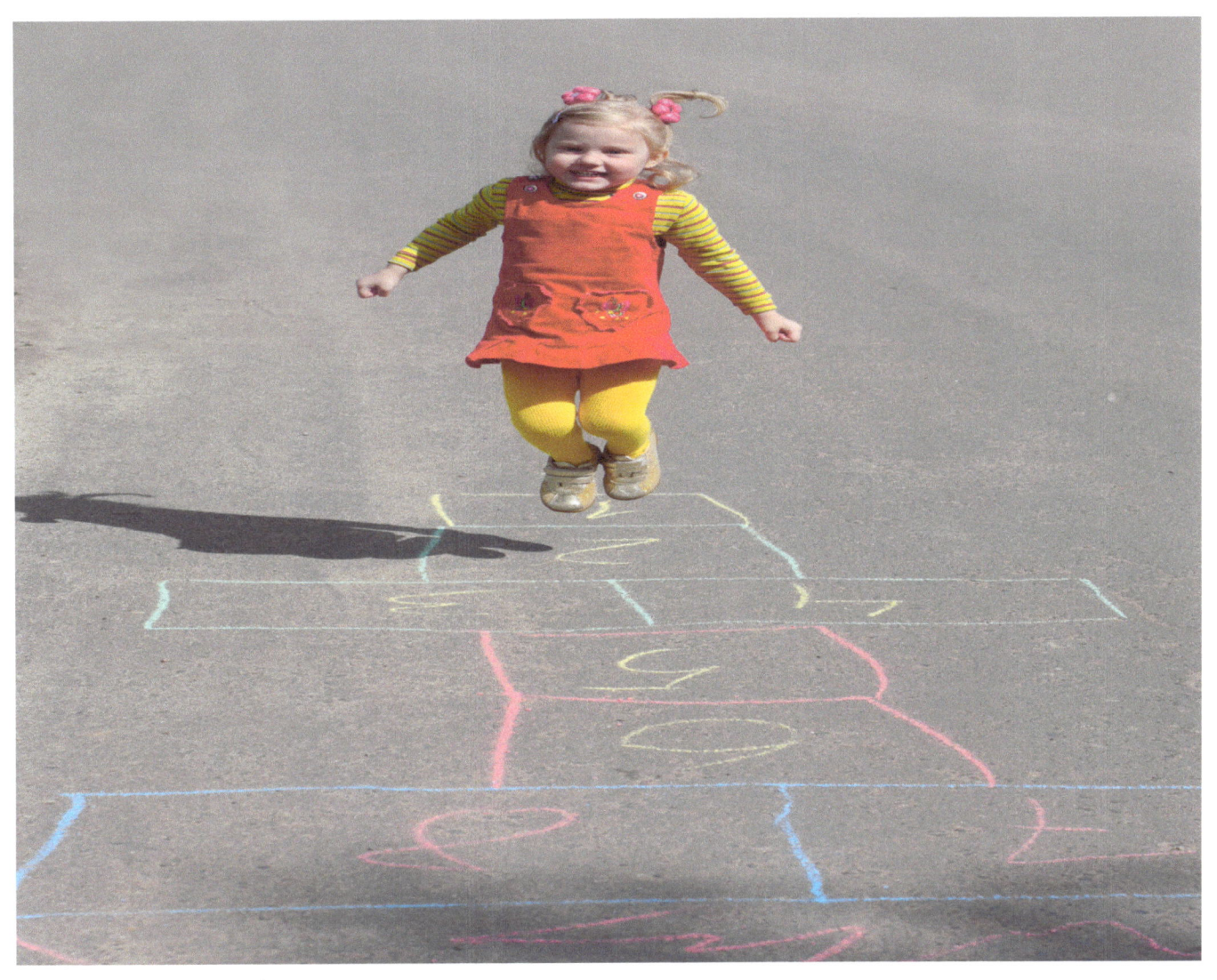

Social Scene 11: This girl is playing hopscotch at the playground by herself. Let's pretend to...

Ask her what her name is...
Tell her your name...
Ask a question or make a comment about hopscotch...
Ask her if you could play together...
Make more comments...
Ask more questions...
Say goodbye politely when you are finished...

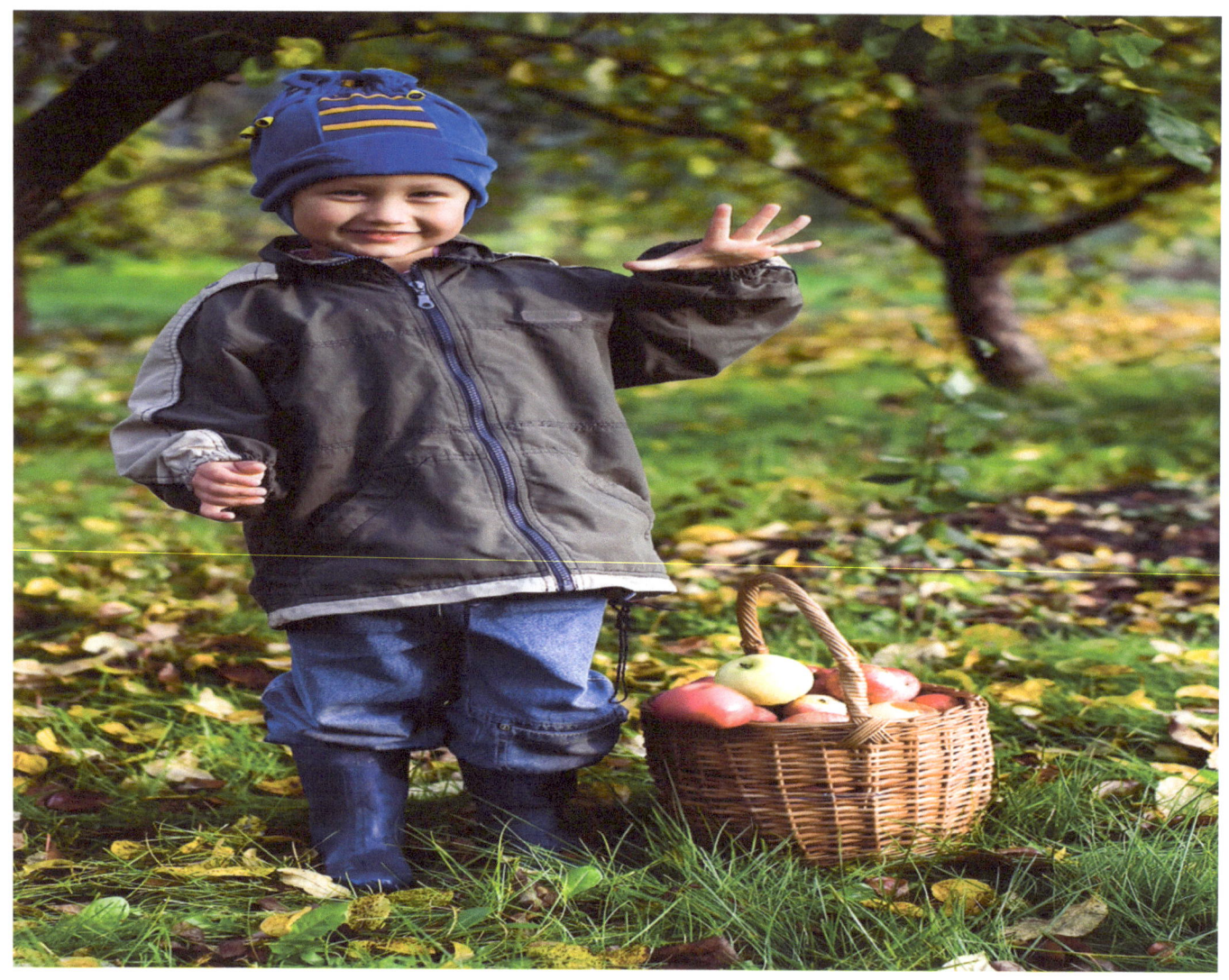

Social Scene 12: This boy went apple picking. He got a whole basket of apples. Let's pretend to...

Ask him what his name is...
Tell him your name...
Make a comment or ask a question about the apples...
Ask him if you and he can pick some apples together...
Make more comments...
Ask more questions...
Say goodbye politely when you are finished...

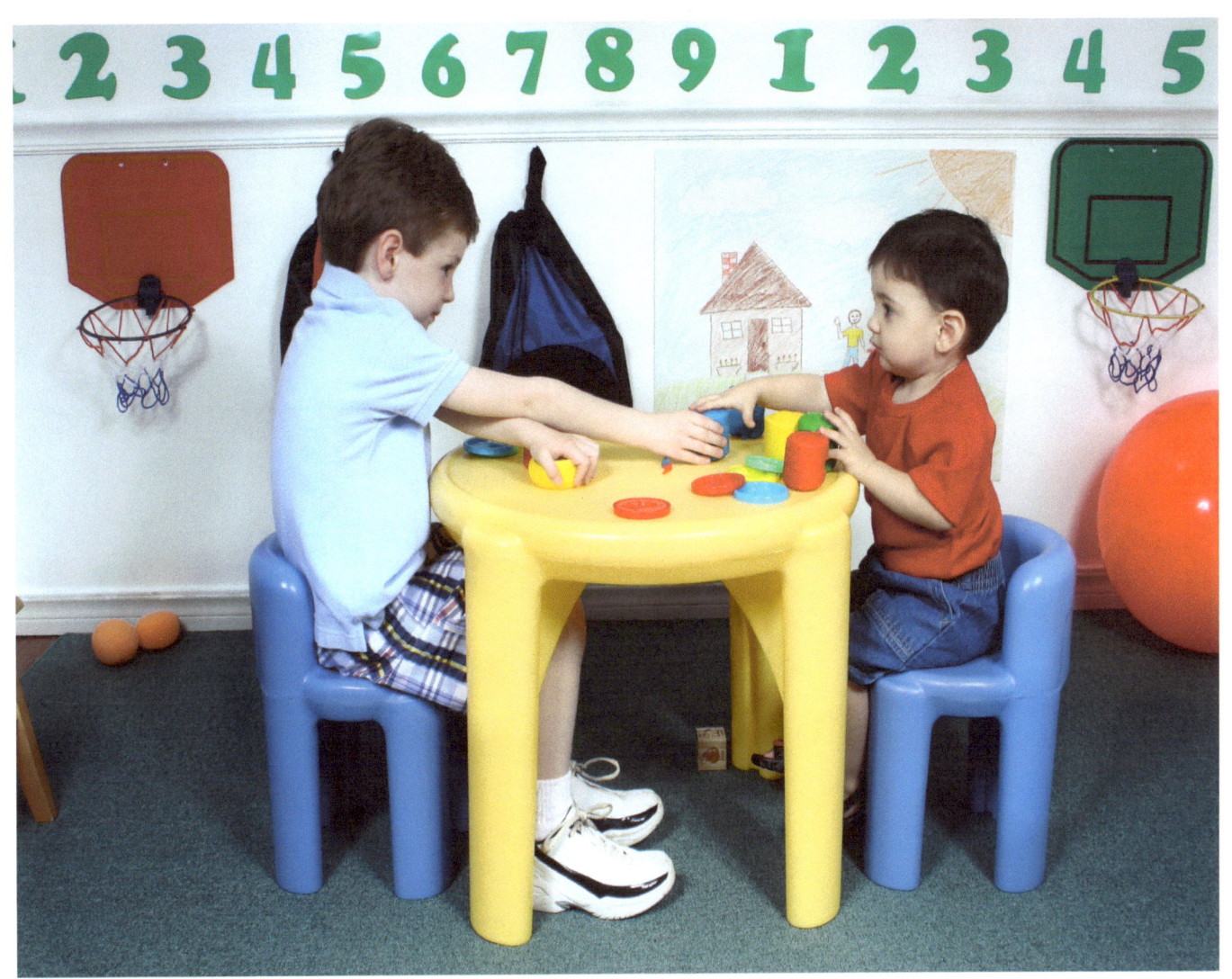

Social Scene 13: These boys are playing with clay together at school. Let's pretend to...

Ask them what their names are...
Tell them your name...
Make a comment or ask a question about clay...
Ask them if you can play with them...
Make more comments...
Ask more questions...
Say goodbye politely when you are finished...

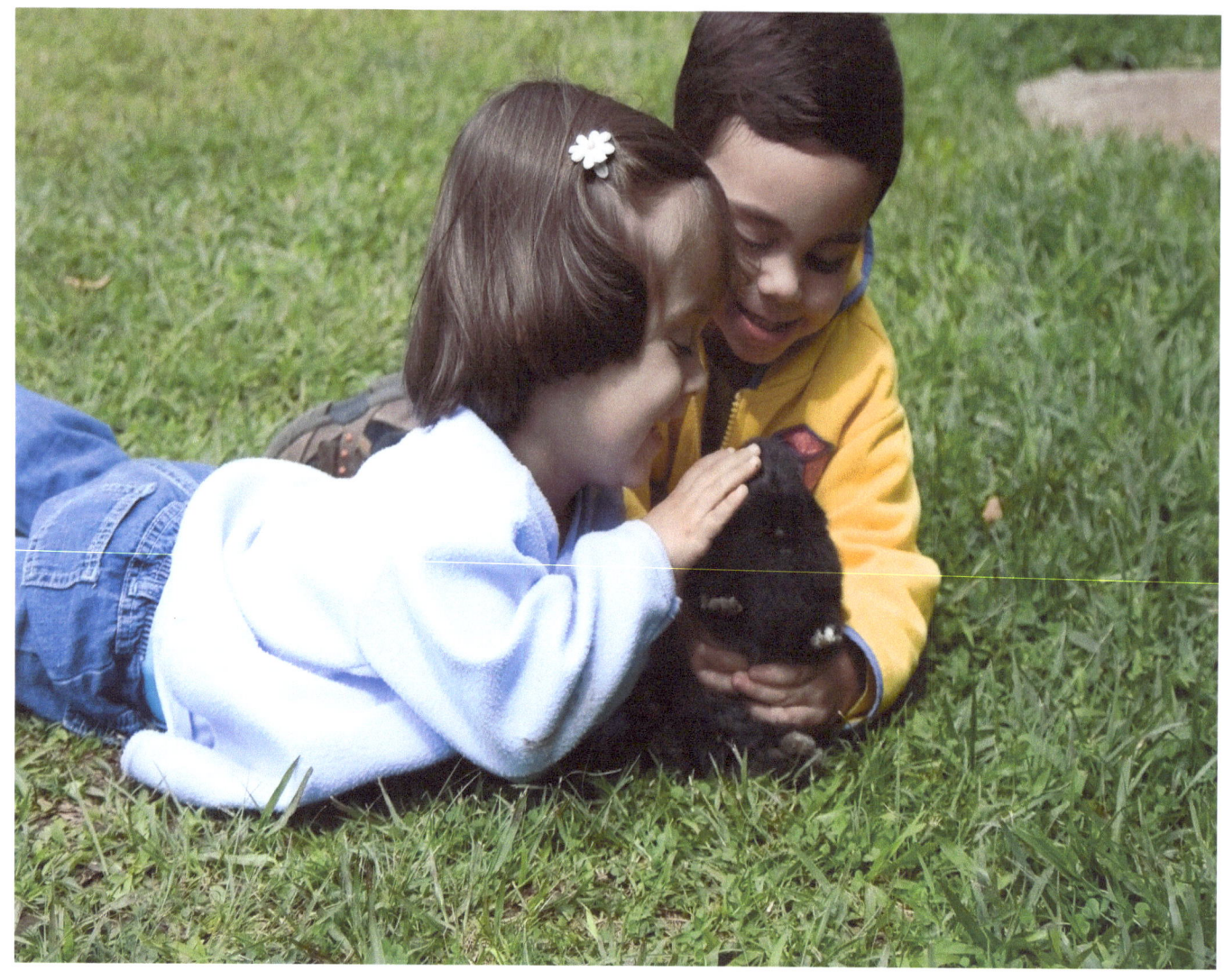

Social Scene 14: This brother and sister are playing with their pet rabbit at the park. Let's pretend to...

Ask them what their names are...
Tell them your name...
Make a comment or ask a question about the rabbit...
Ask them if you can pet the rabbit...
Make more comments...
Ask more questions...
Say goodbye politely when you are finished...

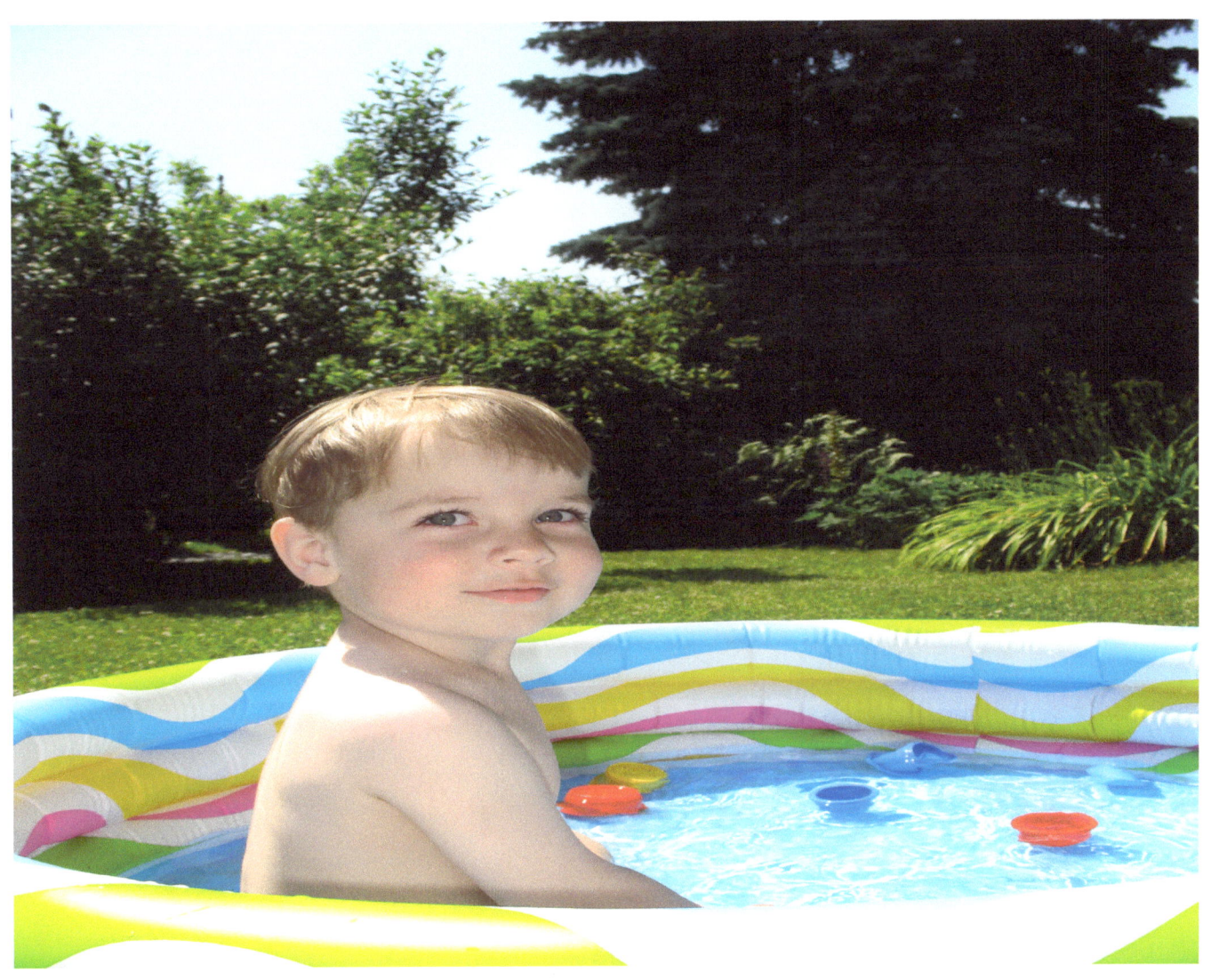

Social Scene 15: This boy is playing in his pool in the backyard. You have not met him yet. Let's pretend to...

Ask him what his name is...
Tell him your name...
Make a comment or ask a question about the pool...
Ask him if you can play inside the pool...
Make more comments...
Ask more questions...
Say goodbye when you are finished...

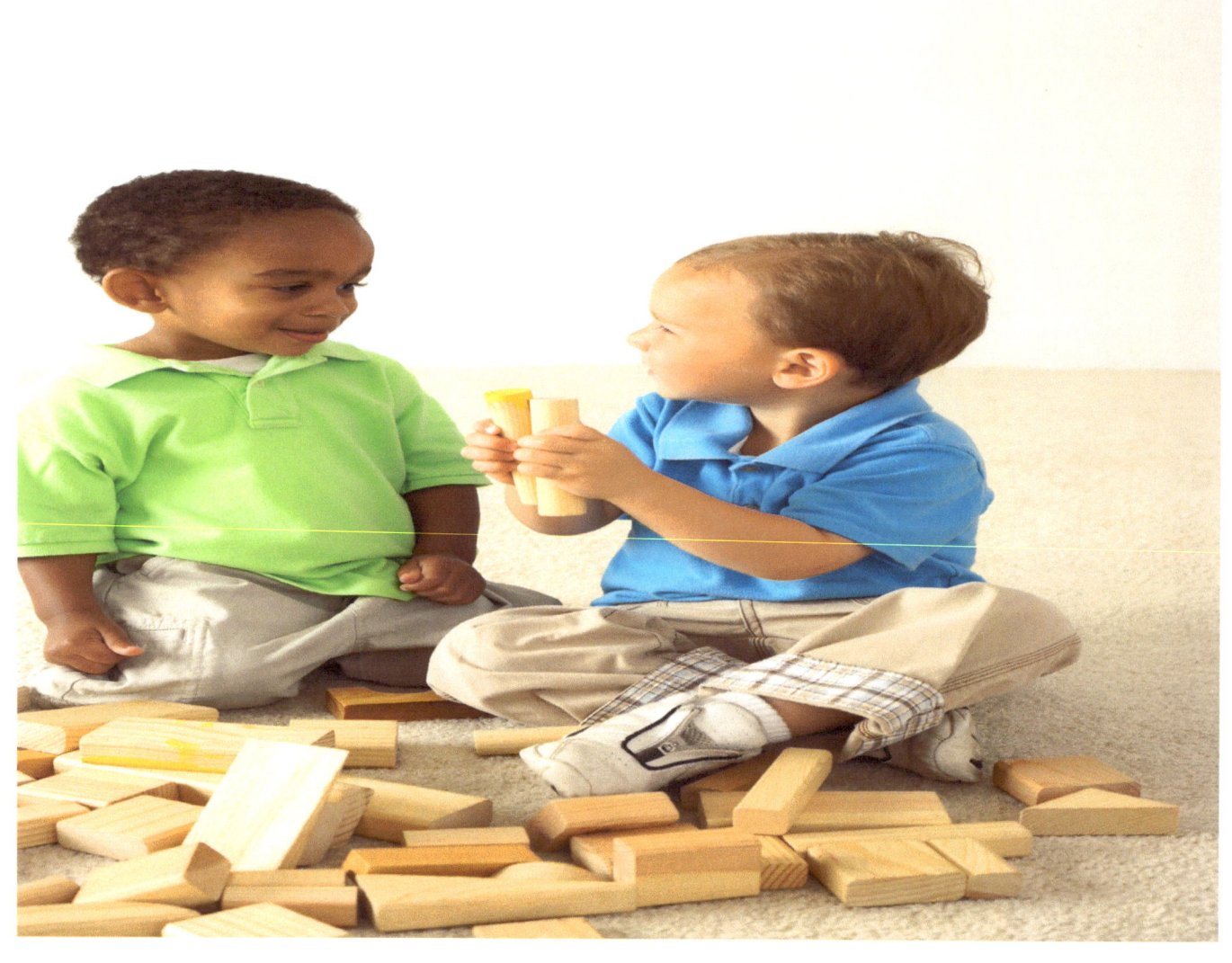

Social Scene 16: These two boys are playing with blocks at school. Let's pretend to...

Ask them what their names are...
Tell them your name...
Make a comment or ask a question about the blocks...
Ask them if you can play with them...
Make more comments...
Ask more questions...
Say goodbye politely when you are finished...

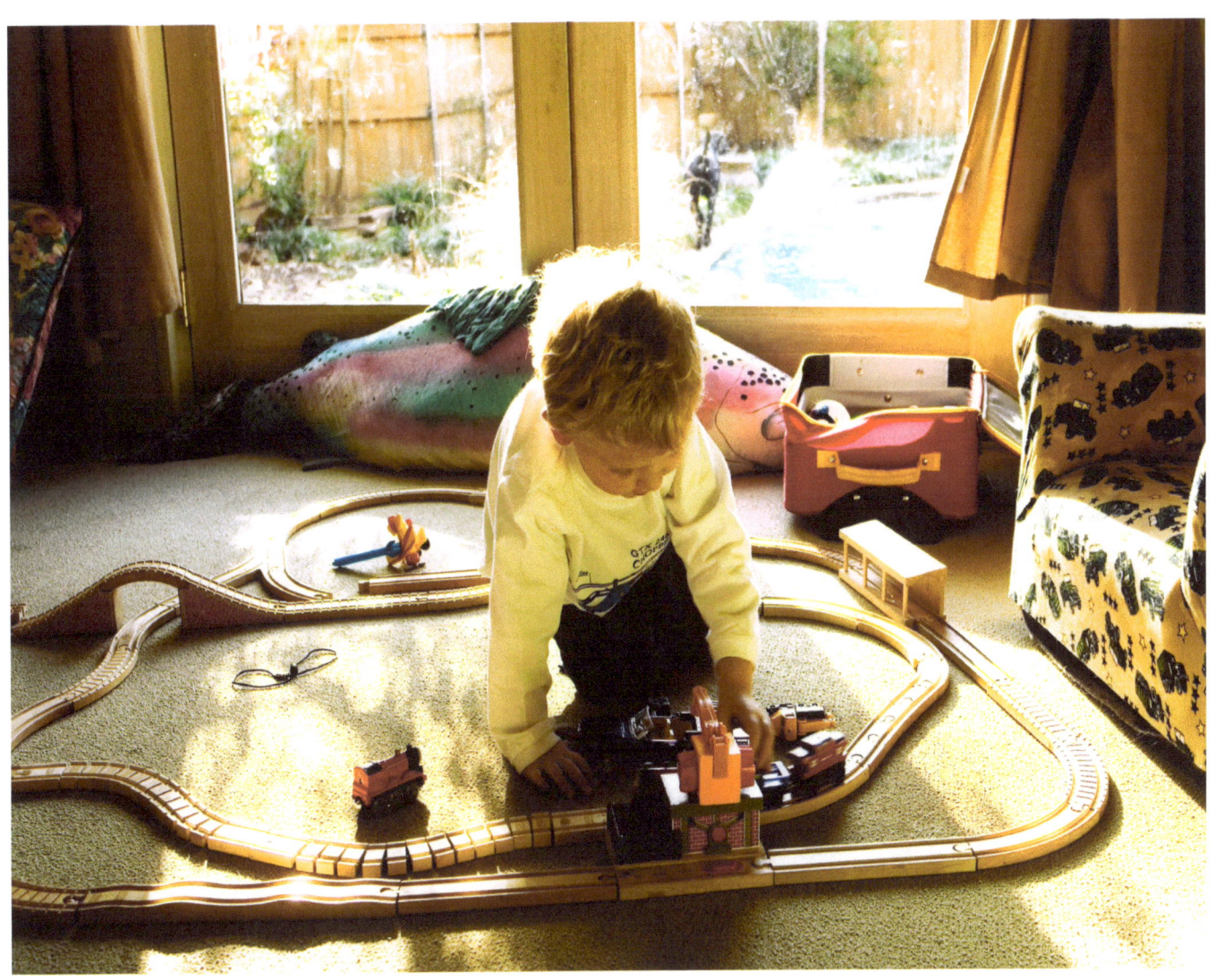

Social Scene 17: This boy is playing with his trains at home. You are visiting but have not met him yet. Let's pretend to...

Ask him what his name is...
Tell him your name...
Make a comment or ask a question about his trains...
Ask him if you and he could play with the trains together...
Make more comments...
Ask more questions...
Say goodbye politely when you are finished...

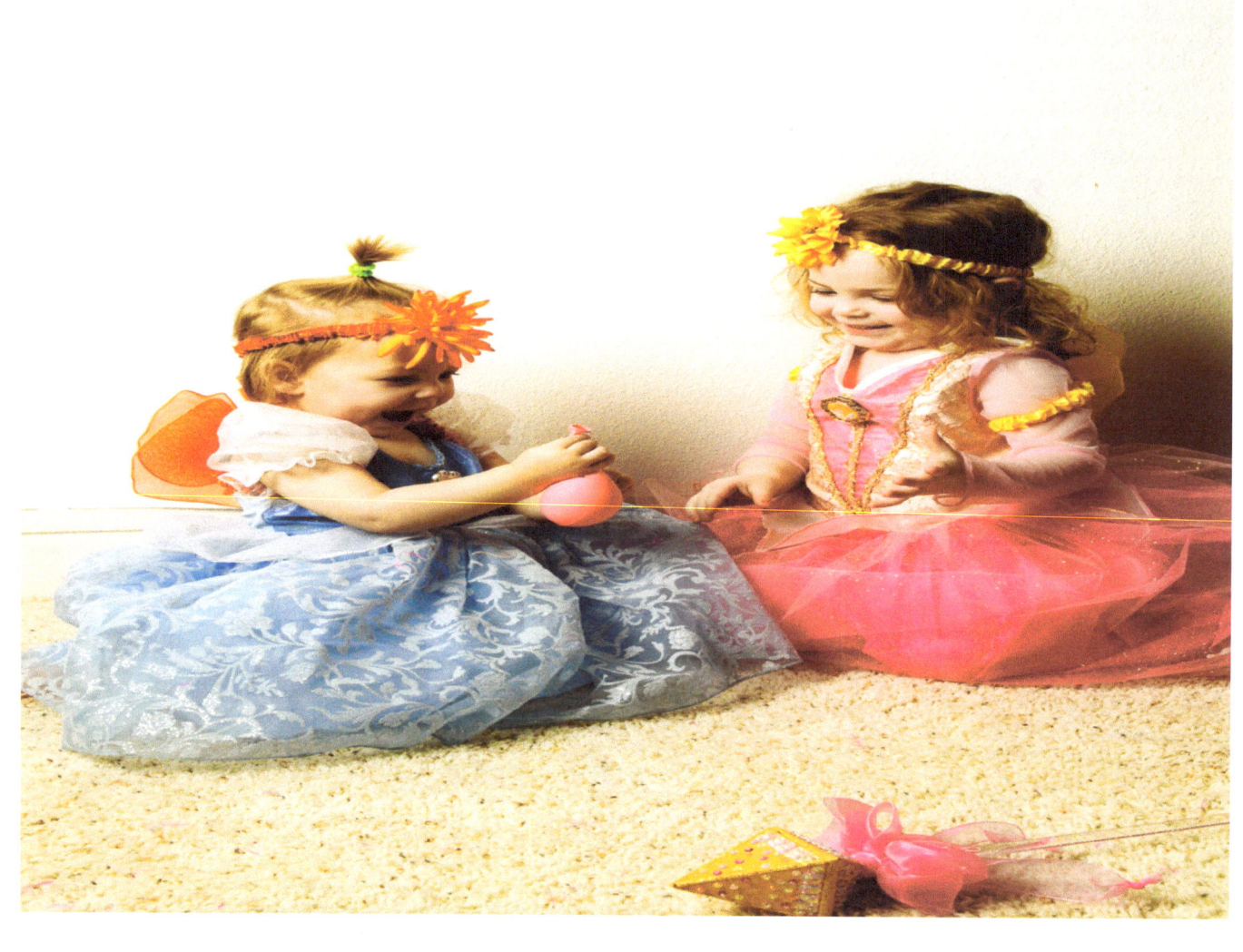

Social Scene 18: Two girls are playing in costumes. They are pretending to be princesses. Let's pretend to...

Ask them what their names are...
Tell them your name...
Make a comment or ask a question about their costumes...
Ask them if you can play with them...
Make more comments...
Ask more questions...
Say goodbye politely when you are finished...

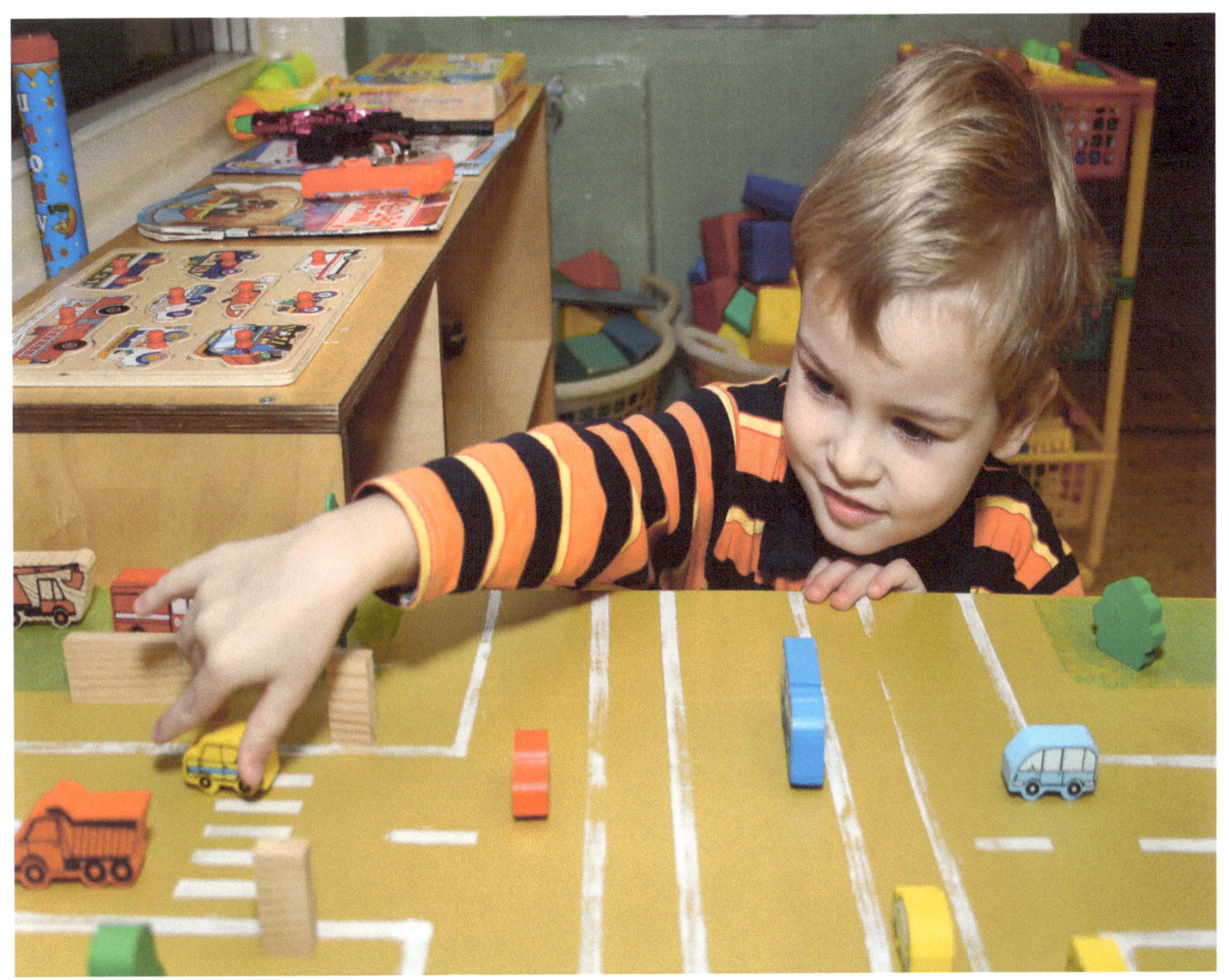

Social Scene 19: This boy is playing with cars and trucks at school. Let's pretend to...

Ask him what his name is...
Tell him your name...
Make a comment or ask him a question about the vehicles...
Ask him if you could play together...
Make more comments...
Ask more questions...
Say goodbye politely when you are finished...

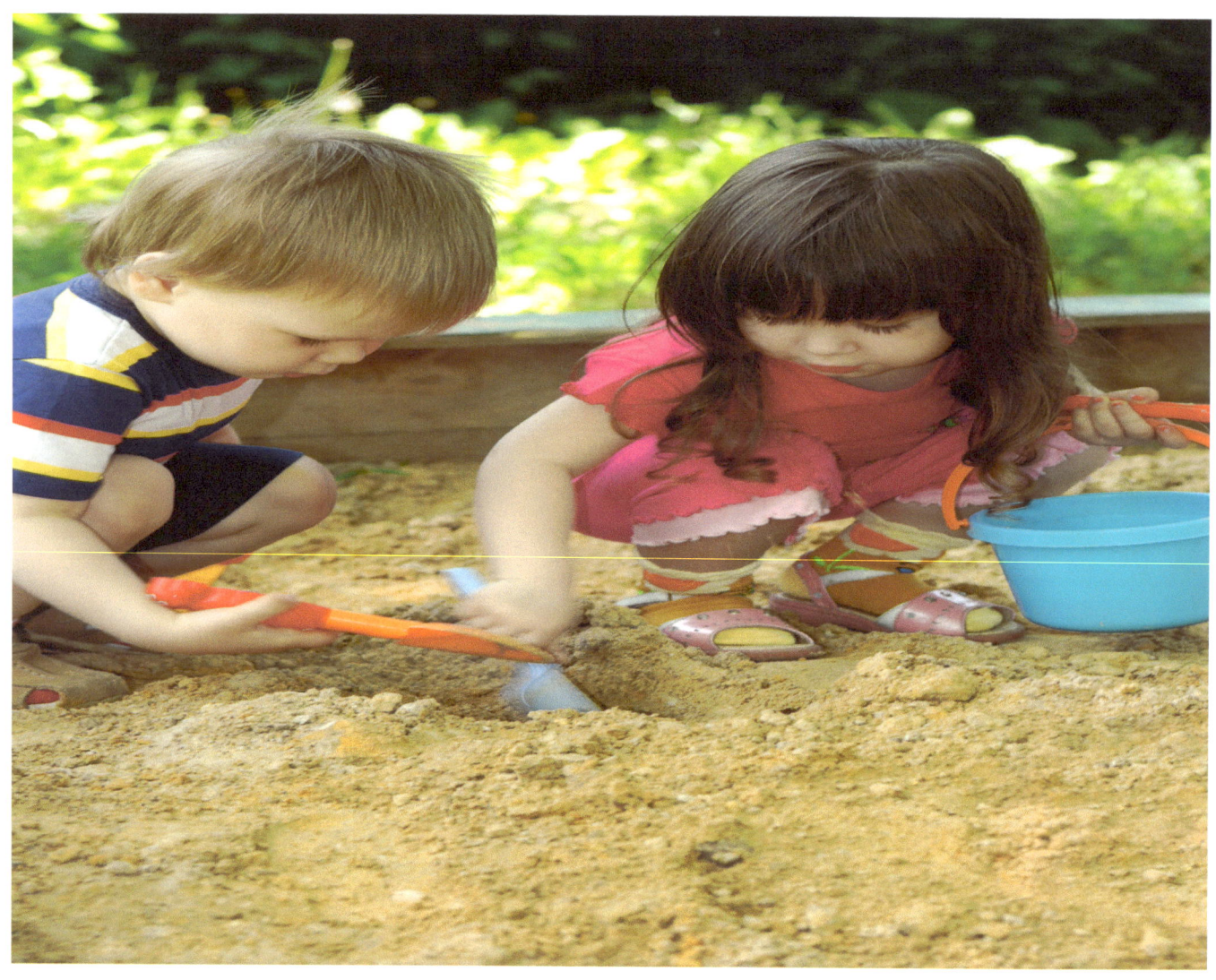

Social Scene 20: This boy and girl are playing next to each other in the sandbox at the park. Let's pretend to...

Ask them what their names are...
Tell them your name...
Make a comment or ask a question about the sandbox or toys...
Ask them if you could play with them...
Make more comments...
Ask more questions...
Say goodbye politely when you are finished...

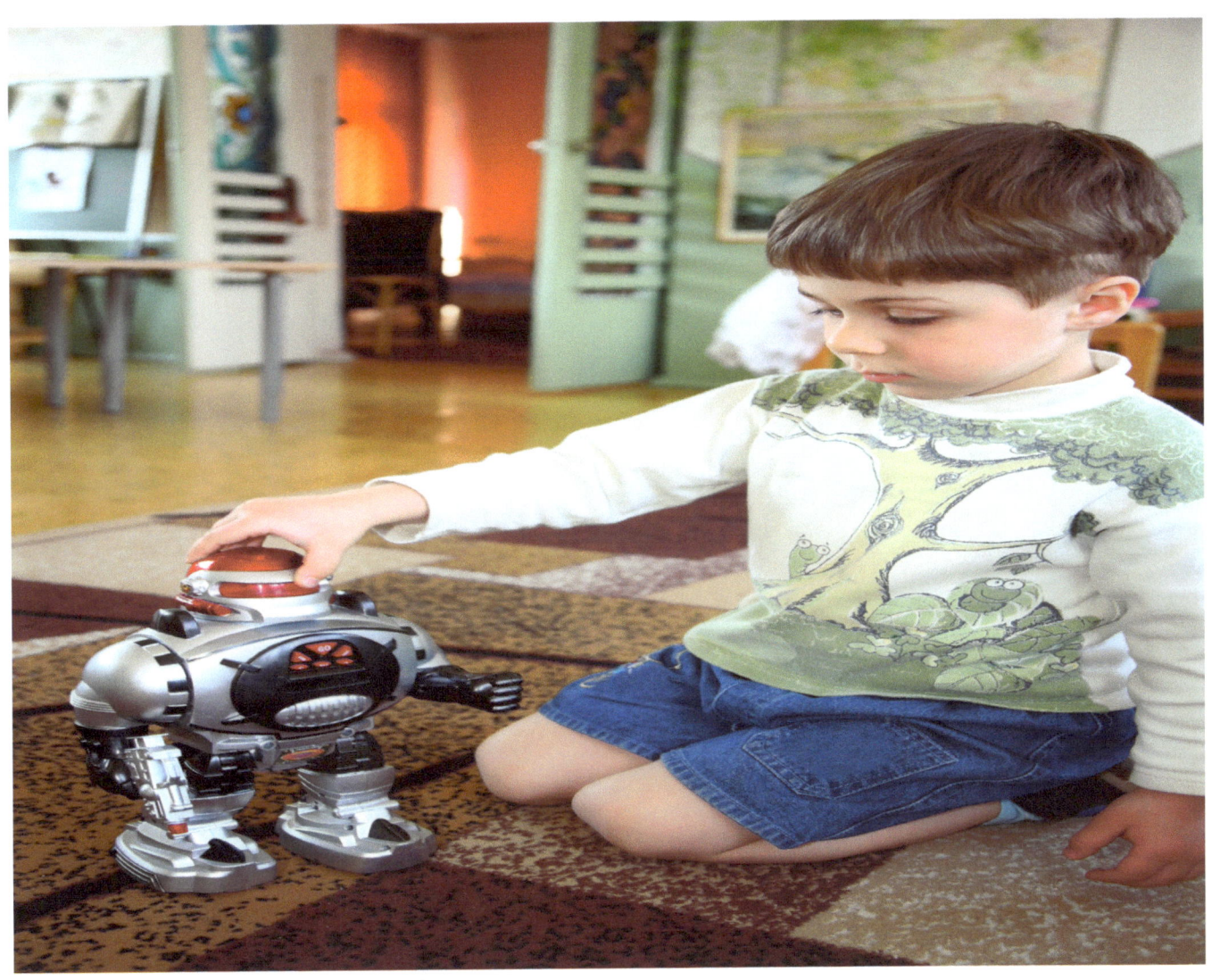

Social Scene 21: This boy is playing with a new toy robot he got for his birthday. Let's pretend to...

Ask him what his name is...
Tell him your name...
Make a comment or ask a question about the robot...
Ask him if you and he could play together...
Make more comments...
Ask more questions...
Say goodbye politely when you are finished...

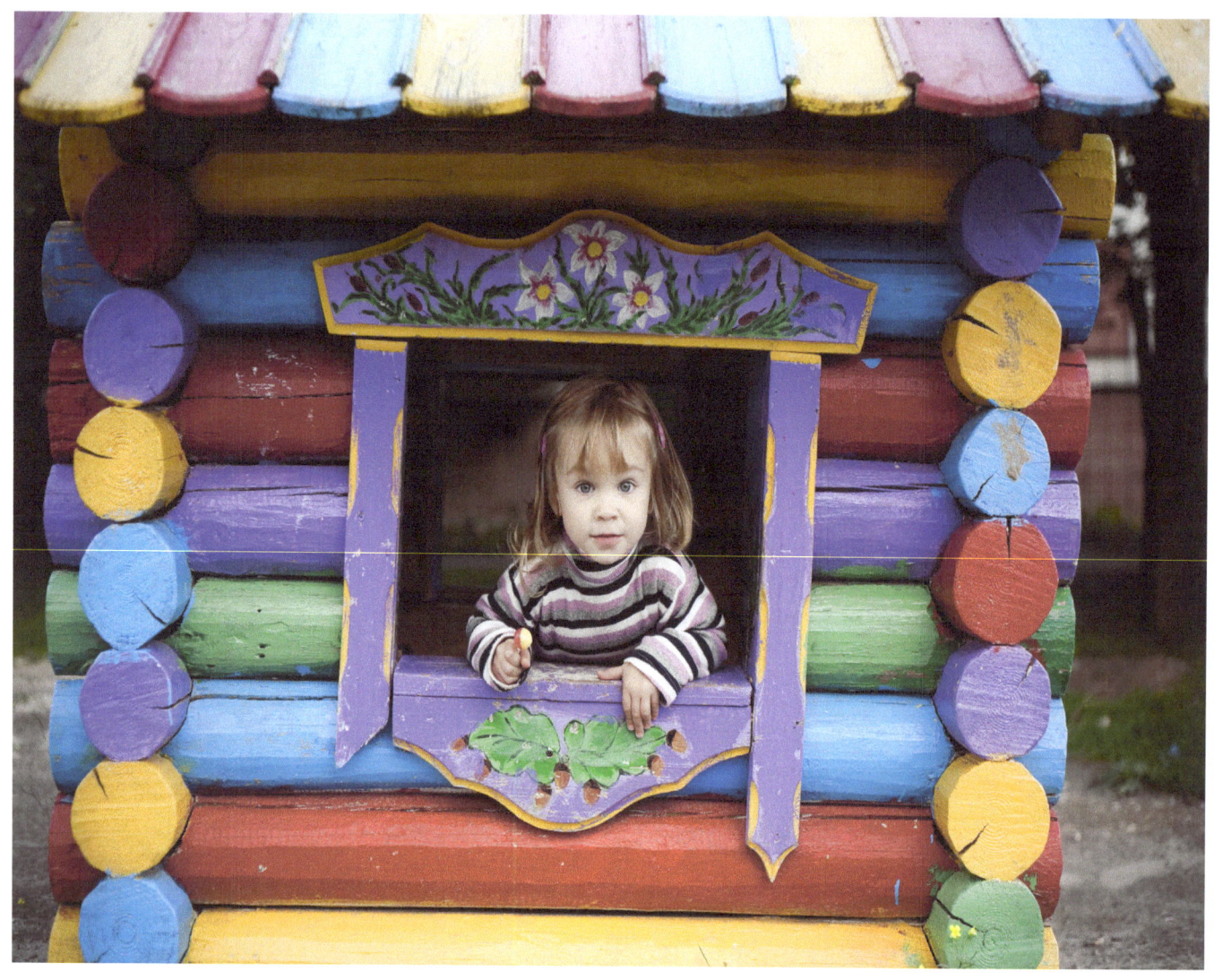

Social Scene 22: This girl is playing in a doll house at a storybook park for children. Let's pretend to...

Ask her what her name is...
Tell her your name...
Make a comment or ask a question about the house or park...
Ask her if she would like to play with you...
Make more comments...
Ask more questions...
Say goodbye politely when you are finished...

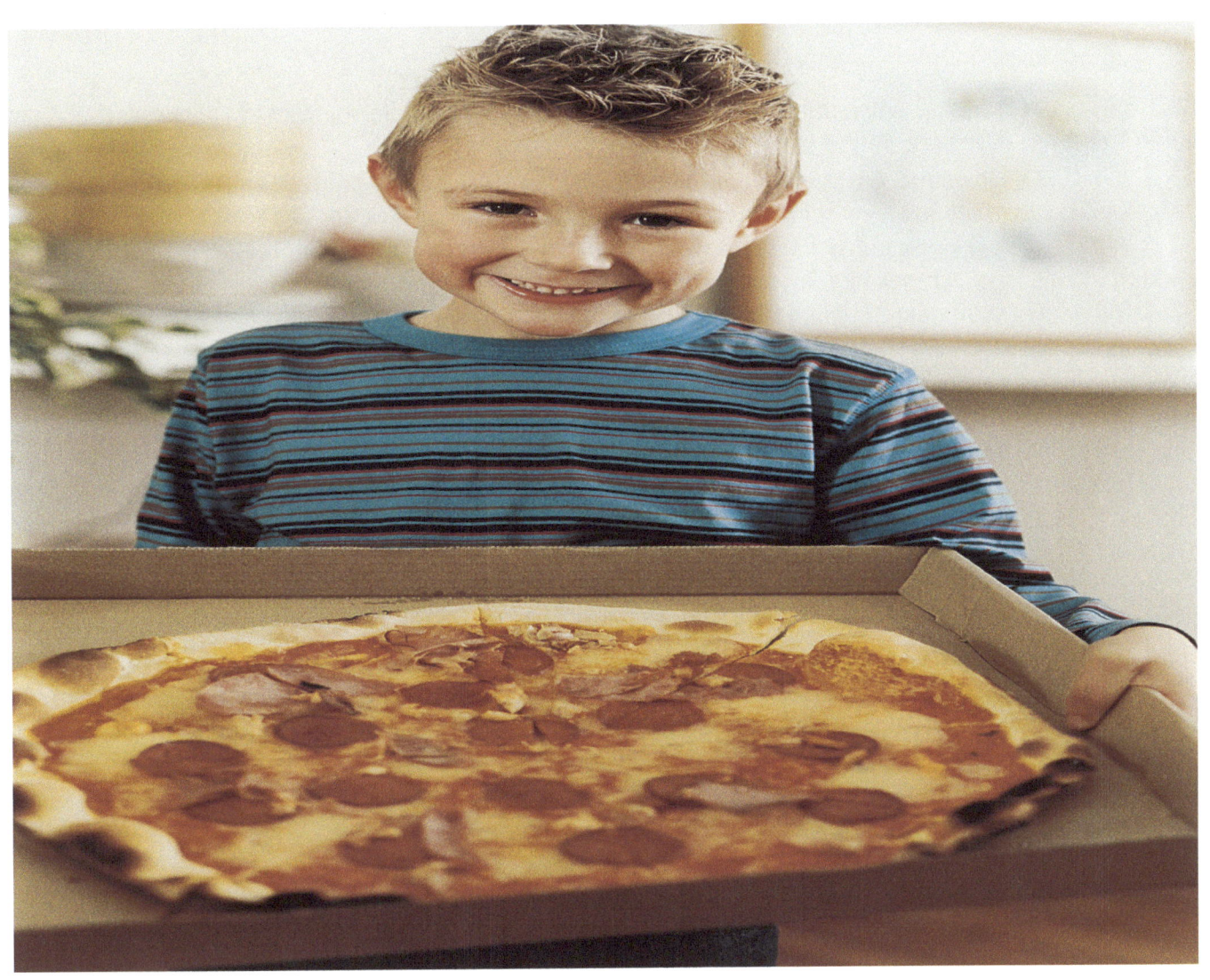

Social Scene 23: This boy is giving away pizza at a pizza party. Let's pretend to...

Ask him what his name is...
Tell him your name...
Make a comment or ask a question about the pizza...
Ask him if you could have some pizza...
Make more comments...
Ask more questions...
Say goodbye politely when you are finished...

Social Scene (SS) Sample Responses

SS 1: What's your name?, My name is ..., There's so many balls in here, Do you want to play together?, I'm going to bounce over here, Do you want to play catch?, See you later

SS 2: What is your name?, My name is..., Nice painting, Do you want to paint together?, What are you painting?, I want to paint my pet hamster, I want to paint my sister, See you next time

SS 3: What are your names?, My name is..., Swings are fun, Do you want to play together?, Can I use this swing?, I can push you if you like, Nice meeting you, bye

SS 4: What are your names?, My name is..., Those bubbles are cool, Can I try to blow some too?, I can make lots of bubbles, Watch me, How many bubbles do you think you can make?, I'll count the bubbles, Nice meeting you both, Bye

SS 5: What is your name?, My name is..., Awesome dogs, Can I pet them?, Can I play with them?, They are fun, I have a pet dog too, What are their names?, Which one is a girl or boy?, Nice meeting you, Bye

SS 6: Hey, what are your names?, My name is..., Nice soccer ball, Can I play with you both?, I like soccer, I'll kick the ball, Do you live nearby?, How often do you come here to play?, This is fun, Well, nice playing with you, Thanks, Bye

SS 7: Hi, what is your name?, My name is..., I really like this slide, Do you want to play together?, I will race you to the slide, Who is going first next?, Do you play here often?, Do you live nearby?, I live pretty close, Nice meeting you, Hope to see you again sometime, Bye

SS 8: Hi, what's your name?, My name is..., Nice gingerbread house, They taste good too, Can I decorate some cookies with you?, What color should I use for the hair?, Can we eat them after?, I love cookies, Thanks for the cookies, See you again sometime, Bye

SS 9: What's your name?, My name is..., Cool jeep you have, Are you going to let it go down the slide?, Can I try it too?, Oh, it's going to crash, Can we do it again?, I have a jeep at home, I love jeeps, Thanks for letting me play with it, See you later, Bye

SS 10: What's your names?, My name is..., That's a nice birthday cake, Are we going to play tag later?, I hope we get to play tag in the backyard, You have a nice house, When are you opening your presents?, Thanks for inviting me to the party, Bye

SS 11: Hi, what's your name?, My name is..., I never played hopscotch before, Want to play together?, You just jump on the letters really fast?, This is fun, You're good at this, Thank for playing with me, See you later, Bye

SS 12: Hey, what's your name?, My name is..., Wow, you have a lot of apples, Do you want to pick some apples together?, You are lucky, This is fun, Did you eat any apples yet?, How are you going to get them home?, Well, see you next time, Bye

SS 13: Hi, what are your names?, My name is..., Is that clay?, Can I play with some clay too?, I want to make a lizard, What are you making?, That is so cool, Let's do this again sometime, See you later, Bye

SS 14: What are your names?, My name is..., Is that your pet?, Can I pet the rabbit?, I had a pet hamster once, I like goldfish, Do you like goldfish?, I have a fish tank at home, Hope to see you both again, Bye

SS 15: What is your name?, My name is..., Nice pool, Can I come inside the pool?, Is the water cold?, What kind of water toys do you have?, Want to splash around?, This is fun, Thanks for playing, Bye

SS 16: Hi, what are your names?, My name is.., Wow, that's a lot of blocks, Can I play with you two?, I want to build a building, I want to build a bridge, What are you going to build?, That's cool, Thanks for sharing with me, Bye

SS 17: Hi, what's your name?, My name is..., Nice train set, Can I play with the trains too?, I have trains at my house, My trains run on batteries, Which one is your favorite?, Thank for playing with me, Bye

Social Scene (SS) Responses Continued

SS 18: What are your names?, My name is..., Are you both princesses?, Can I pretend with you too?, I want to be a king or queen?, Do you have a crown for me?, I am royal, I have my own castle?, Where is your castle?, Can we go there?, Thanks for playing with me, See you later, Bye

SS 19: Hi, what's your name?, My name is..., What are playing with?, Can I play with you?, I like trucks a lot, Can you pass me a truck?, Which one is your favorite?, Thanks for playing, See you later on

SS 20: What's your names?, My name is..., Did you find anything in the sand?, Can I play with you both?, I need a shovel, Can I borrow this shovel?, Are you making anything?, I want to make a fishpond, I need some fish, I'll pretend the pebbles are fish, This is fun, Nice playing with you, Bye

SS 21: What's your name?, My name is..., Nice robot you have there, Can I play with you?, I have a white robot at home, It can talk, Does your robot talk?, Let's make him go over there, It is so funny, Thanks for letting me play with it, See you again, Bye

SS 22: What's your name?, My name is..., This doll house is neat, Do you want to play together?, Do you come here often?, This park is great, I come here every Sunday, How often do you come here to play?, Well, nice meeting you, See you again, Bye

SS 23: What is your name?, My name is..., Wow, lots of pizza, Can I have some?, I eat pizza at least once a week, How often do you eat pizza?, Can I have two slices?, This is yummy!, Thanks, Nice meeting you, See you again sometime, Bye

Data Suggestions:

Keep data of individual progress by keeping records of children's social communication responses, social awareness levels, perception levels, and role-playing abilities. Mark on graph paper and calculate the changes in those numbers throughout time.

Child's Name:
Date: Social Scene Number:

Examples of Data Targets and Information

Number of social conversation turns with modeling____
Number of social conversation turns without modeling___
Number of social conversation turns with prompting____
Number of social conversation turns without prompting____
Number of appropriate spontaneous responses____
Number of inappropriate spontaneous responses____
Number of grammatically correct responses____
Number of grammatically incorrect responses____
Average mean length of utterances____
Change from previous dates (increase or decrease in appropriate spontaneous responses)____
Other data scales and observational tools:
Social Awareness Scale (relates to the social scene) level (rate from 1 beginner to 5 expert)____
Social Perception Scale (perceives the social scene accurately) level (rate from 1 beginner to 5 expert)____
Ability to Role-play Scale level (rate from 1 beginner to 5 expert)____
Digital recorder and video observations comments:

www.ingramcontent.com/pod-product-compliance
Lightning Source LLC
Chambersburg PA
CBHW041503220426
43661CB00016B/1243